HEALING WITH FRUIT

Using Fruit to Heal Yourself Naturally

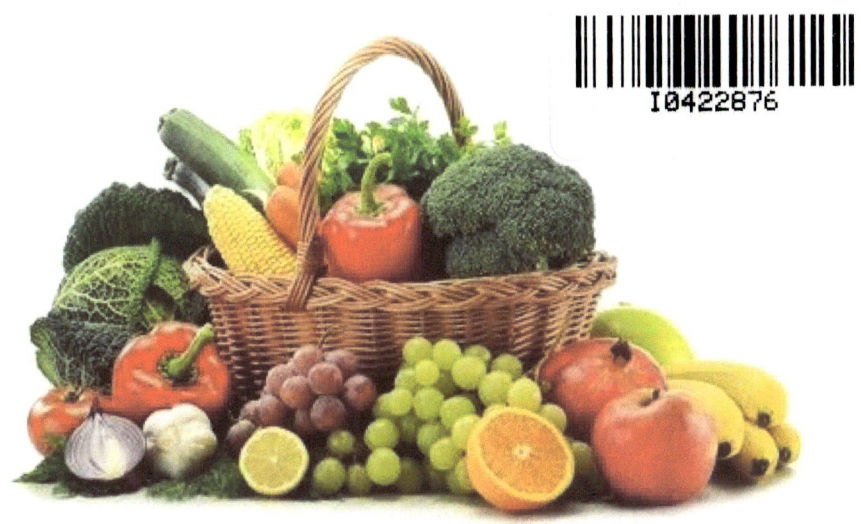

I0422876

Dueep Jyot Singh

Healthy Living Series

Mendon Cottage Books

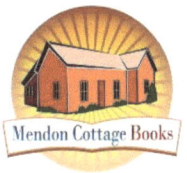

JD-Biz Publishing

Our books are available at

1. Amazon.com
2. Barnes and Noble
3. Itunes
4. Kobo
5. Smashwords
6. Google Play Books

Table of Contents

Introduction

Many naturopaths know that vegetables and fruits are excellent healers, but most of these timeworn remedies have been lost, just because we are so used to popping pills and taking short-term shortcuts in healing ourselves.

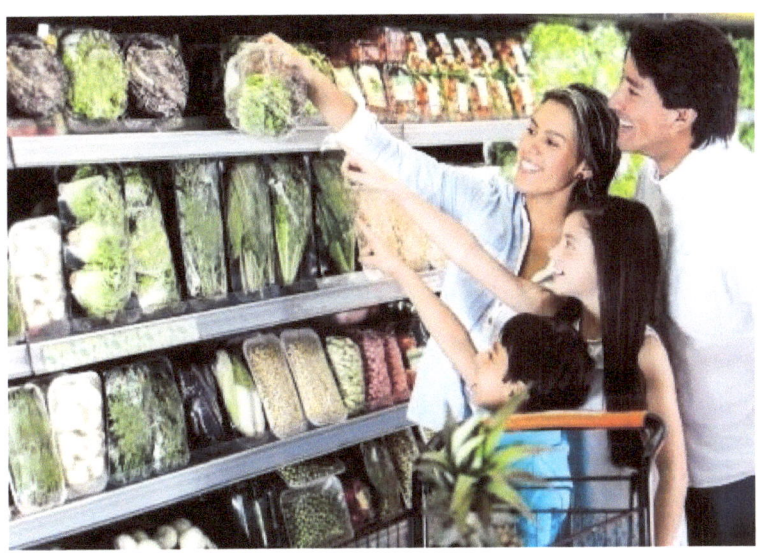

Nature has made our body so adaptable, taking into view its bio – physiological makeup that fruit, vegetables, spices, and other natural products are extremely beneficial in helping to heal natural ailments.

This book is going to tell you all about these natural remedies which have been practiced down the millenniums by Wise Men down the ages, to help heal and cure problems. These remedies were also supported with natural products like milk, butter, and yogurt along with honey to provide the body with its deficiency of vitamins, minerals and carbohydrates, which may have been the possible causes of deficiency diseases.

Down the ages, men have been using ginger, onions, garlic, radishes, lemons, apples, carrots, different vegetables, herbs, spices, and milk products like yogurt, butter, and milk to provide man with nourishment as well as healing natural materials. However, these remedies were also supplemented with lots of fruit, which would help in helping keeping him healthy. So pick out your favorite fruit and see how it is going to cure you of common ailments.

Apple

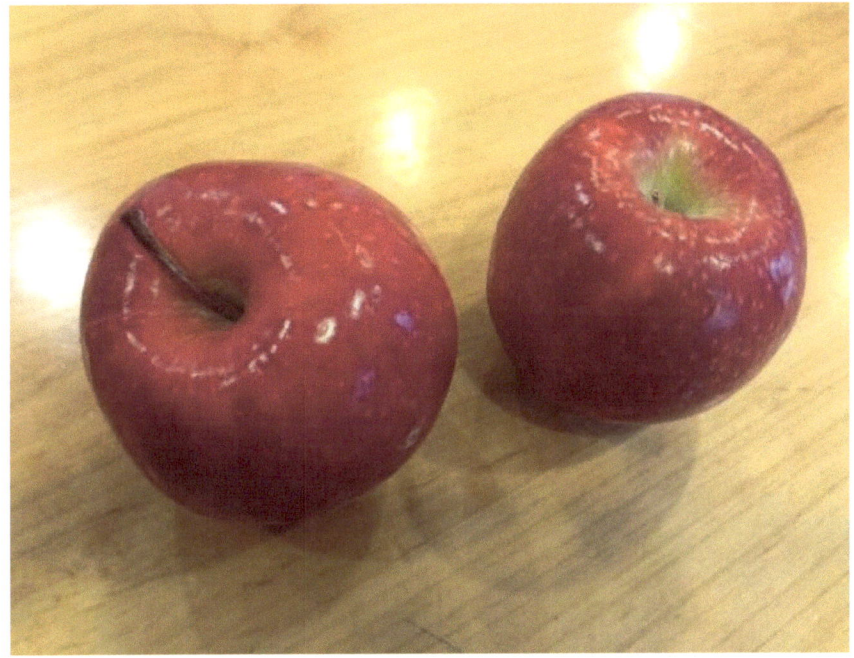

As we are going to start right at the very beginning with the clichés of an apple a day keeps the doctor away, let us look at the time tested remedies, which this delicious fruit provides us. An apple a days going to provide you with lots of energy, purify your blood, and strengthen your digestive system. It prevents problems in the kidney and the liver and also helps you if you are suffering from gout.

Cough

If you are suffering from a chronic cough, just take out the juice of an apple, fresh and filter it. Now add a little bit of rock candy to this juice and drink it first thing in the morning, before eating anything else, or brushing your mouth. You are going to find your cough disappearing before the week is over.

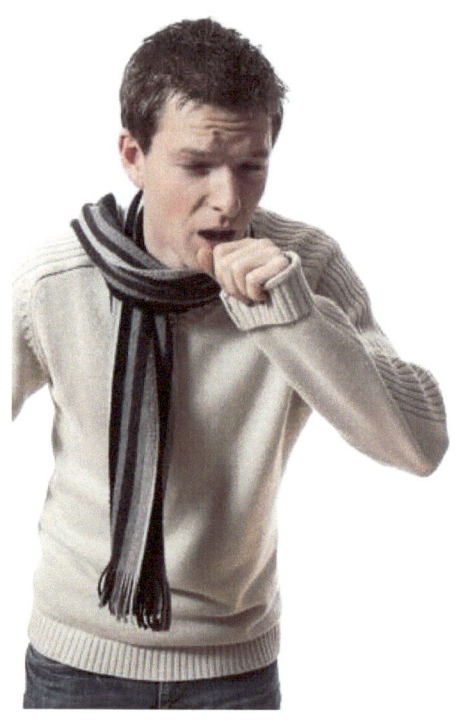

Headache

Headaches are normally caused through stress, or as a signal that there is something wrong in the system somewhere. They can also be caused due to eyestrain. Apples are excellent to get rid of chronic headaches. In fact, this remedy was told to me by one of my herbalist friends, who knew that I suffered from migraines. But it was too late, because my migraines had been cured, naturally, with the passing of time.

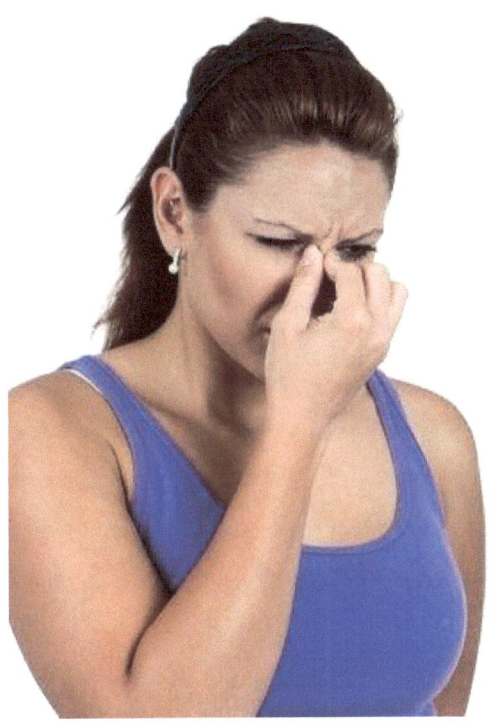

So if you find yourself in such a situation, every day, here is how you are going to get rid of the most tiresome headache, especially when it appears that the onset of the morning, and does not leave you till late at night.

Just chop up one or two apples after peeling them. Do not throw the peel away. [You can always eat the peels later mixed with a little bit of salt and pepper. They are extremely good roughage for your digestive system.]

Mix a little bit of salt in these bite sized pieces, and eat them first thing in the morning, before you eat anything else. This eating first thing in the morning has since ancient times been considered to be the best way of healing yourself. You did not wash your mouth out before hand.

The ancients considered the saliva in a mouth just freshly woken up from sleep was very healing. So when you ate something or drank something, that healing saliva would benefit you. So whenever I say first thing in the morning in my future remedies, it means exactly that.

If you are like me, and cannot eat anything or drink anything without brushing your teeth first, washing your face or having a bath – as taught as little children – you may want to try out this alternative healing idea of eating or drinking something on a "stale" mouth.

So eating these apples, with a little bit of salt, for the next few days is going to get rid of every vestige of headache, even chronic ones and migraines. I wonder why researchers have not bothered giving patients this natural remedy to get rid of chronic headaches, but then how would they sell their drugs if they did so?

Redness in the Eyes

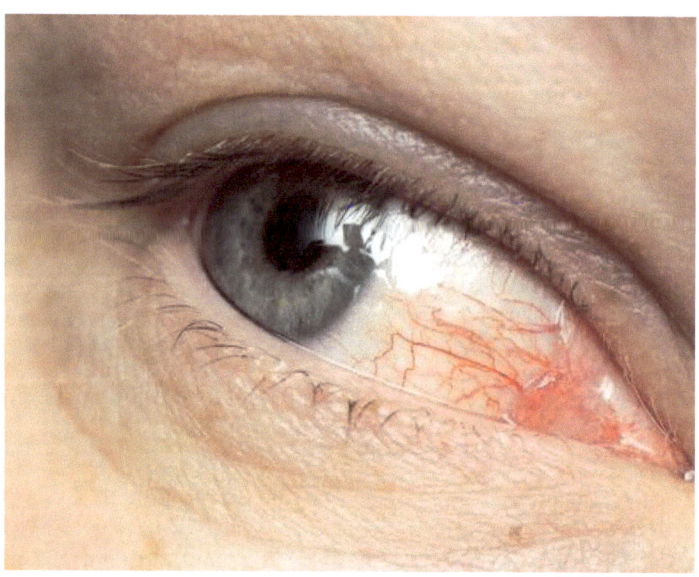

Redness in the eyes can be caused due to strain, lack of sleep, and even possibly an infection in the eyes. Wash your eyes with warm water. Carefully pat them dry. Then peel an apple, and apply the peel on that affected area. Now, bandage this peel with a muslin cloth, bandage, and allow it to rest for half in hour. Not only is this going to refresh your eyes, but it is also going to get rid of any sort of pain and strain.

In fact, instead of eating the peel, you may want to apply it on your eyes as a refreshing cooling "tonic".

Nausea and Sunstroke

When we were children, we were given fresh apple juice with a little bit of salt in it every morning with breakfast, so that we never suffered from nausea in the summer. Also, we did not suffer from sunstroke or any dehydrating effects of sun worshiping, to which, alas, we were badly addicted.

In fact I remember during the summer vacation, when all good children should have been resting at home in the afternoons, the principal of our school complained to our father that we were there, on the building site of the school, which was being repaired, in the burning hot sun, getting in the way of the construction workers.

He could not imagine how anybody in his right senses would want to go out in the sun in the blazing heat of June, and enjoy it. According to him, any normal person would come down with either a headache or a sunstroke or heatstroke. But we never did, because we had apple juice for breakfast, and when we came back home, we were immediately fed a large cooling glass of either fresh lemon juice or freshly made buttermilk.

And so we flourished in temperatures of 38°C (100°F) in the shade, to the great dismay of our elders, especially horrified principals – and never came down with sunstroke or heatstroke.

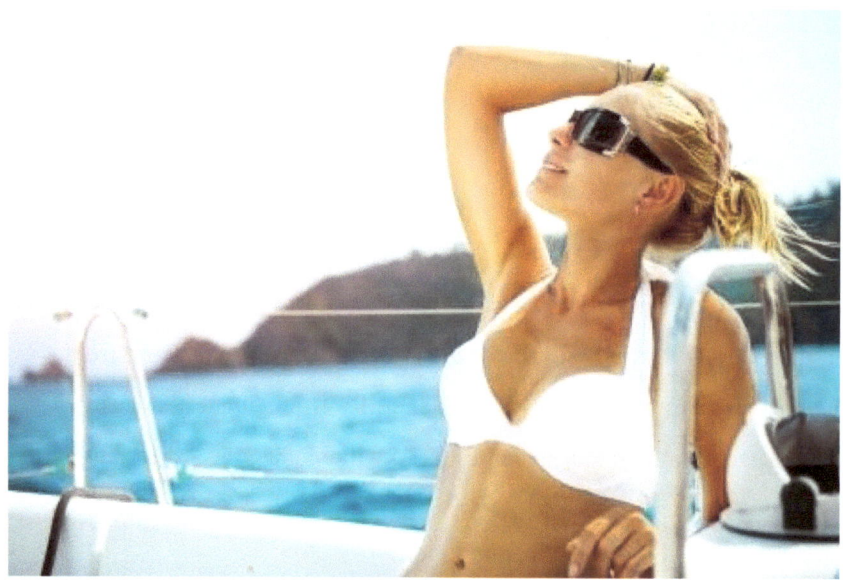

She may be roasting herself well in the sun, but she is going to come down with a headache or possible sunstroke, because she does not have protective headgear.

Mental Health

This remedy was told to me by a doctor, who said that he prevented his elderly parents from suffering from senility just by feeding them a fresh apple, – unpeeled – before any of their meals, and even in their 80s, they were mentally alert and physically healthy. Apart from that, he said that whenever he felt tired, mentally or found that there was a loss of concentration, he just took out an apple from his lunchbox and munched on it.

That immediately made him feel more energetic and his brain felt rejuvenated. In fact I found many of my friends munching on apples and other fruit, during lunchtime, and they were more energetic than the rest of us. So possibly, my Doctor friend does have some thing going there.

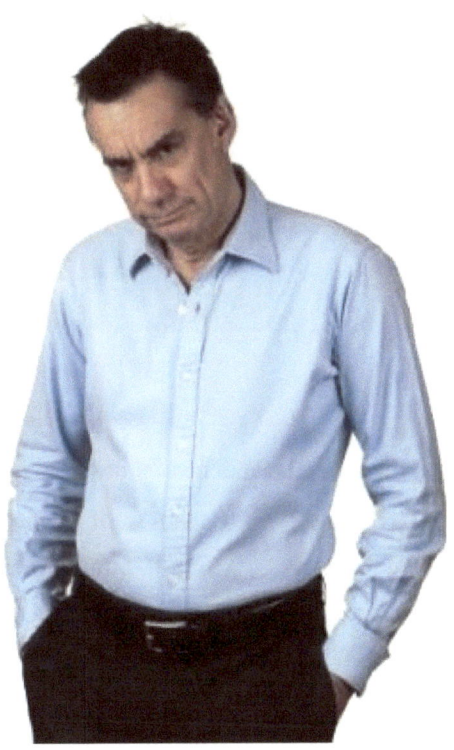

Feeling grumpy, energetic, or just in a bad temper, just because you feel a loss of concentration? Boost up your Apple consumption.

Grapes

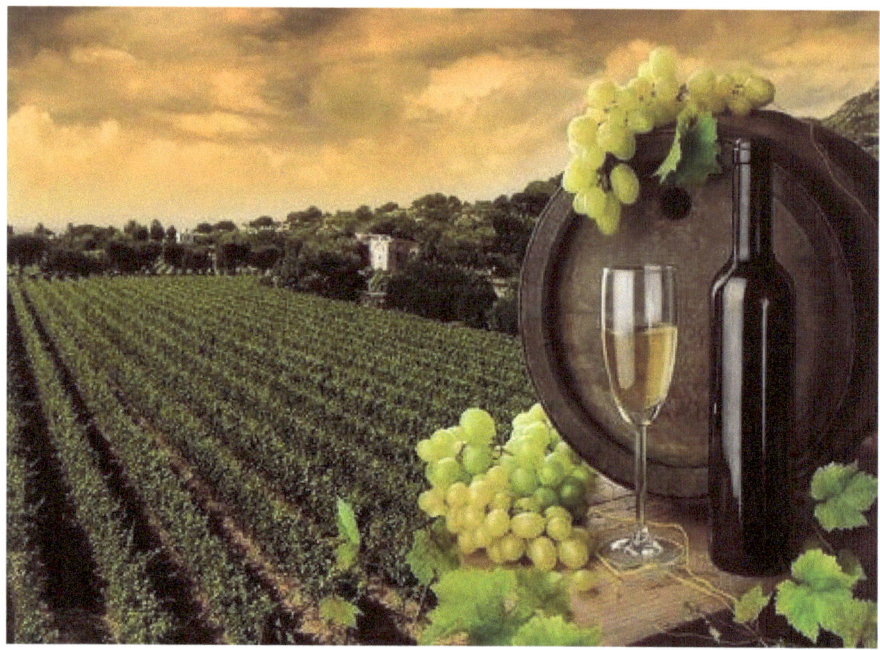

Since ancient times, the grape has been considered to be the fruit of the Gods, especially in Greek mythology, because it purifies the blood, gives you plenty of energy, is nourishing and delicious, and is extremely good for your digestion. It is also good for curing problems of your liver and ailments of the blood.

Liver Ailments

In ancient times, liver ailments were cured with the help of grape leaves. Fresh grape leaves were taken off the grape vine – about 20 g of them, and mixed well with water. A little bit more water was added to it, to make it a grape leaf juice/pulverized grape leaf mixture and this was fed to the patient.

If there was pain in the liver region, it was cured within an hour or so, with just this mixture.

Also, people suffering from bleeding from the mouth, nose, or the urinary passages could be cured well with plenty of grapes, a few at a time, at regular intervals.

Incidentally, grapes have been known since ancient times to cure tumors and cancer. The researchers do not want to admit it, grapes have been used by naturopaths to help prevent cancer from occurring again, especially when the patient is in remission, and also healing him slowly. In fact, my aunt suffered from cancer and had to go through terrible chemotherapy sessions in Paris. She was also clinically declared dead two times, but when she came back the second time, she said to heck with it, she was not going to go through this painful chemotherapy and its equally debilitating side effects.

She came back home, and began her own natural cure sessions, because she was a naturopath. She lived a comparatively healthy existence, without any further attacks of cancer – for the next 28 years on fruit juice, raw vegetables, grapes, and buttermilk, absolutely nothing else. And she died in her sleep 28 years later.

I would not suggest anybody try this option, because doctors are going to be roaring for my blood. But it has been proven that a diet of grapes and only grapes for three months, and then grapes with buttermilk has shown a visible marked improvement in cancer within the year, and healing within the next four years.

Along with this, the only grain that you are going to eat is whole-wheat bread with butter, – if you can get clarified butter, so much the better, and lots of honey and buttermilk. This was considered to be the food of the

Gods, and the ancients ate it every day in large quantities. And they lived for centuries, if we believe what is written in the sacred books and treatises of yore.

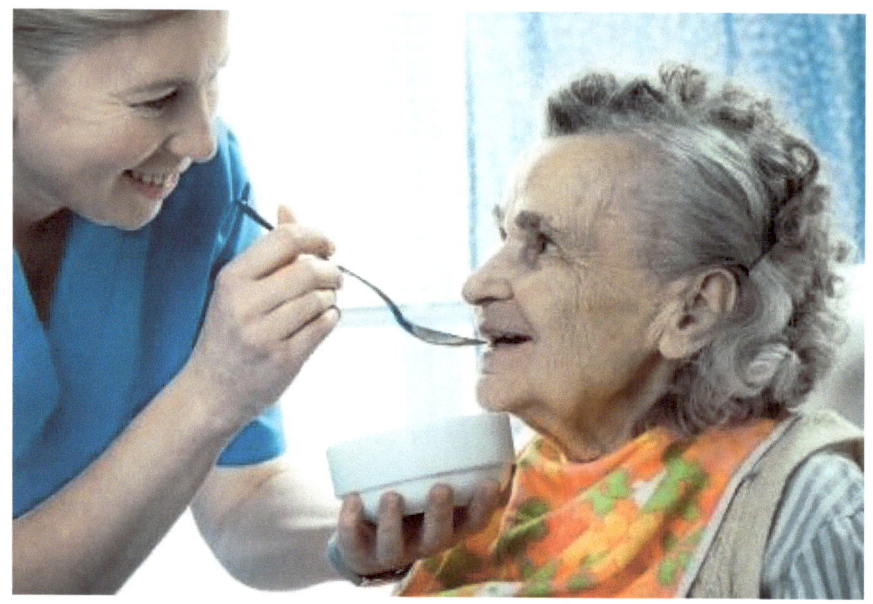

If the elderly are given lots of honey in their diets, they are going to keep healthy and alert.

This is her regime, which she followed strictly. Before she went on a grape diet, she fasted for three days with just grape juice. After that, she started eating as many grapes as she could. But the quantity she ate was never more than 1 pound or more a day.

After three weeks, she began to drink lots of buttermilk along with the grape juice. During this time, she did not eat anything else. And that means that exactly. Only grapes and buttermilk.

This cure took a while, but she began to show marked improvement within the next seven months.

During this cure, she was not given anything cooked – that means cereals, vegetables, or anything else for the first six months.

The first two months, she ate just grapes and buttermilk. After that, she added other fruits to grapes, in order to supplement the mineral and nutritional content. This continued for another one month.

After that, the fourth month, she ate raw vegetables along with grapes and fruit. These vegetables and fruit included tomatoes, green salads, and even dry fruit for energy.

From the sixth month onwards, she began taking cooked food in small quantities and she found herself healthier, and with absolutely no recurrence of the disease.

Urinary Infections

Urinary infections can have other side effects on your health, like headaches and nausea.

I know a lot of people who suffer from chronic urinary infections. They are very miserable. But this can be cured permanently by just taking 50 g of raisins and soaking them overnight. The next morning you are going to crush them with one teaspoonful of roasted cumin seeds powder. Drink this crushed grape/ water/cumin seeds powder down. Try this for one week, and see the urinary system getting rid of all its infections permanently.

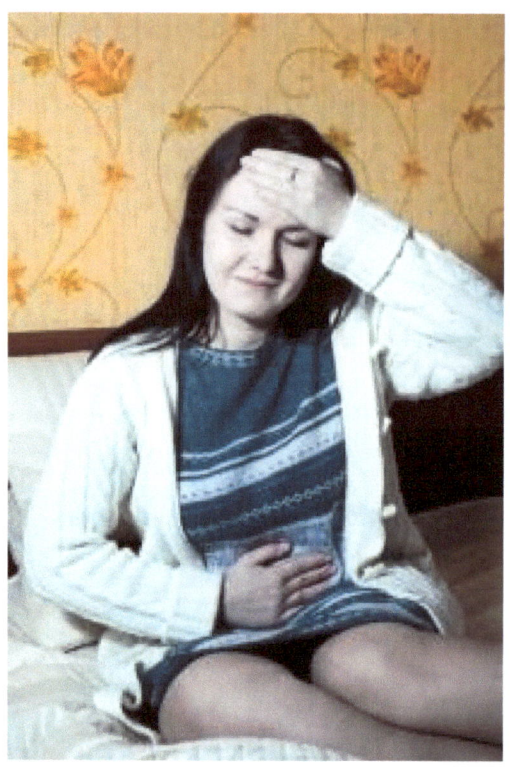

Constipation And Acidity

Constipation and other problems related to bad dietary habits can easily be cured with lots of fresh grape juice. If a baby suffering from constipation, all you have to do is feed him a tablespoon full of fresh grape juice. His system is going to turn normal again.

In the same way, if the babies are fretful because they are teething and feel feverish, just give them a glassful of fresh grape juice morning and evening and you are going to have happy, healthy babies without any of that continuous grizzling tormenting your eardrums.

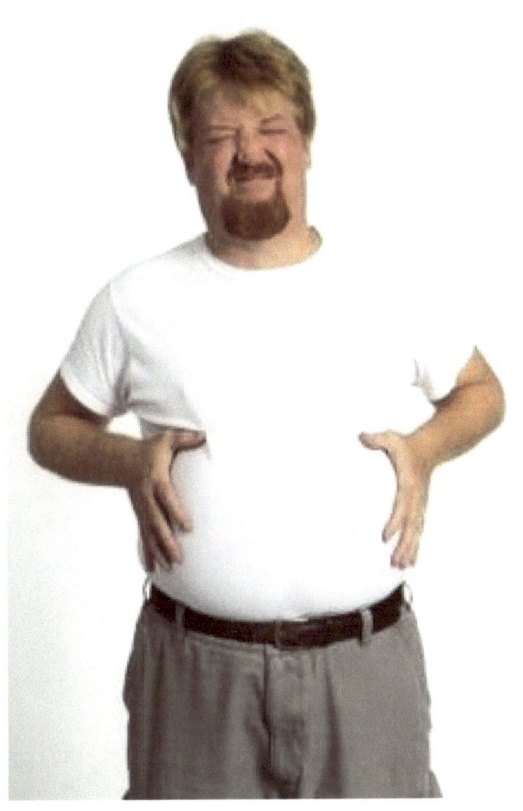

If you are suffering from acidity mix up equal measures of pomegranate juice and grape juice. This is an excellent cure for acidity and even nausea.

Grapes for Eye Ailments

In ancient times, when people didn't bother much about hygienic surroundings, children and adults suffered very often from eye problems, including itching eyes and pain in the eyes. That was when the near proximity of a grape plant was considered to be a godsent.

If you have your eyes paining, all you have to do is take some raw green grapes and crush them. Just put two drops in each eye, in the morning and repeat this every day, for the next three days to find your eyes cured of this pain.

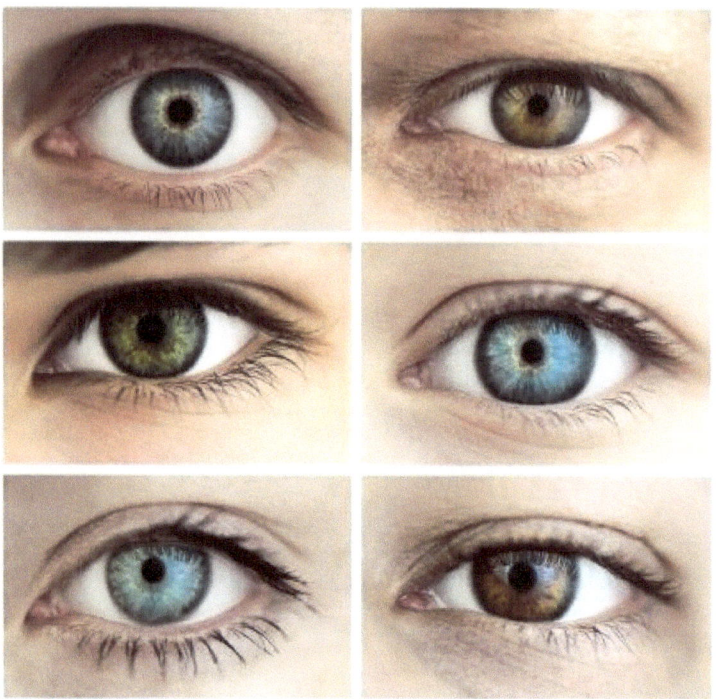

Irritated Eyes

Also, if you find yourself rubbing your eyes very often due to irritation, just take some fresh juice of grapes, and put them on the fire to grow even more concentrated. This concentrated very powerful grape juice is then placed in a glass bottle. Before you go to sleep, you are going to dip an applicator in this juice and put the juice in your eyes. This gets rid of the irritation. It also makes your eyelashes grow really well.

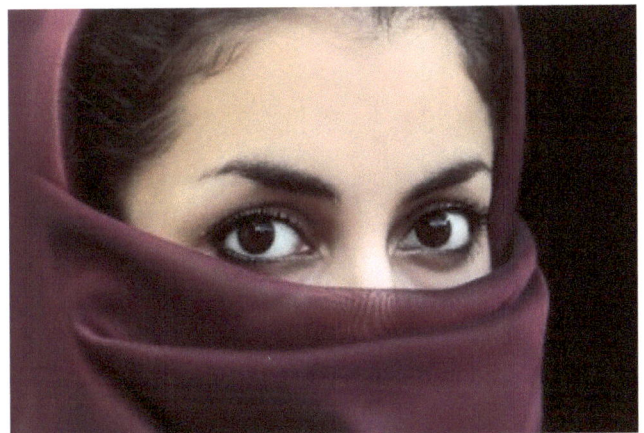

In ancient times, people used to use an applicator, normally made up of silver to apply kohl or surma – as called in Egypt and other Middle Eastern countries, – to their eyes at night. By the time they woke up in the morning, there was just enough of kohl left on their eyes, to give it a beautiful look and color throughout the day.

Even today, if you see Egyptian wall paintings, you are going to see that both men and women outlined their eyes with blue kohl. A silver applicator and bottle is of course going to be extremely rare to find, and of course exorbitantly priced, but you can find kohl bottles made up of other metals like brass, and other alloys online, at bargain prices.

A couple of years ago, I met some friends, from the Northwestern Frontier region – Afghanistan and beyond – and I was surprised to see the eyes of all the men lined with dark powdered Surma. I was under the impression that it was a totally feminine beauty adornment. But they did not seem to be at all conscious about it and took this part of grooming to be a part of their normal lives.

Chronic Fever and TB

People suffering from chronic fever should be given plenty of fresh grape juice. In olden times, people suffering from tuberculosis were given lots of grape juice, with honey so that they did not suffer from weakness. Funny enough, this cure has been disregarded in a large number of natural healing centers, where people go to cure themselves of chronic fever and also in tuberculosis sanitariums.

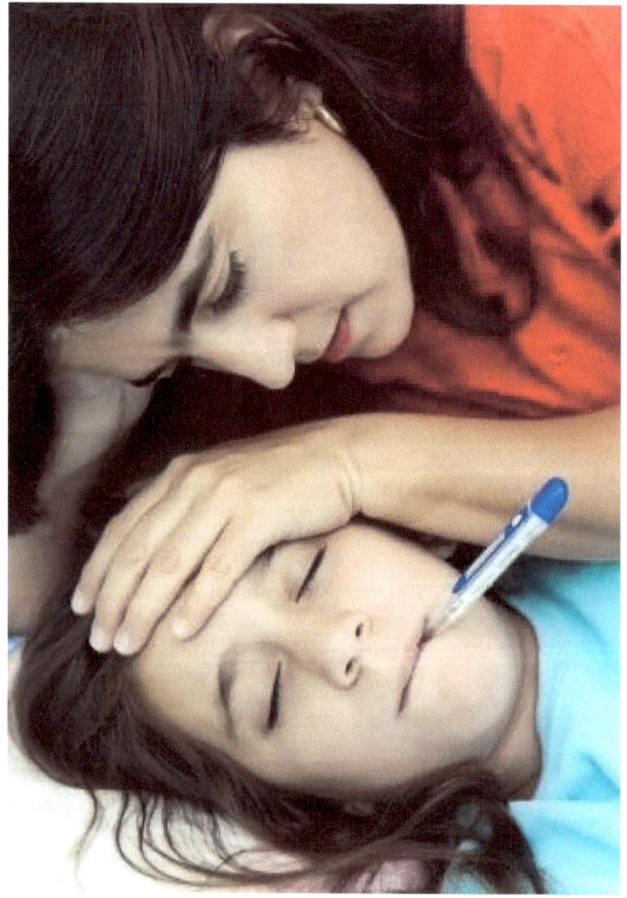

It will take a little while for you to cure itself with grape juice for chronic diseases; that is why you need patience. It is not going to give you a visible effect within 24 hours. The normal time taken to cure serious chronic diseases is one month. Within the six week, you are going to find a visible bettering of the patient's condition.

You are going to start this cure by eating 100 grams of grapes, early in the morning, once a day. Then start increasing the quantity of the grapes that you can eat, so that in the next five days, you can manage anywhere between 1 pound of grapes to more. Children can eat these grapes according to their own capacity.

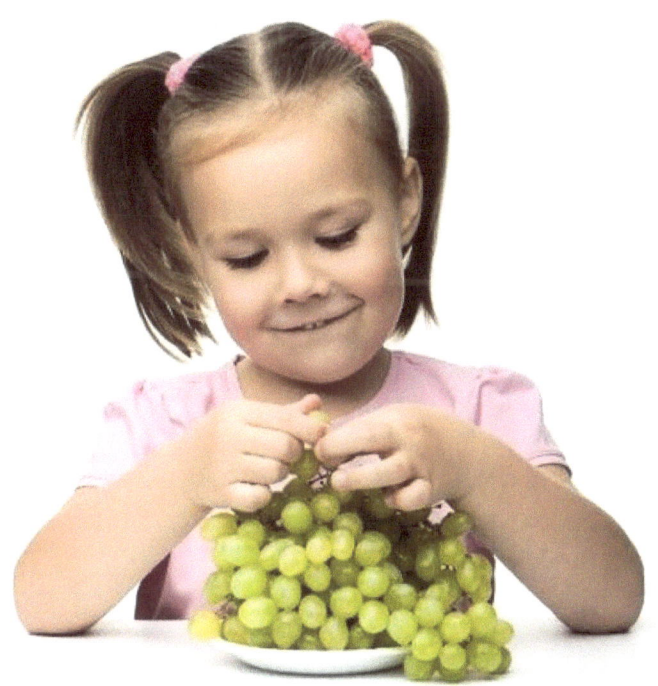

When you find yourself improving, do not stop eating these grapes suddenly. Begin to lessen the quantities of the grapes being eaten until it matters out completely. By then you will have cured yourself.

Oranges and Lemons

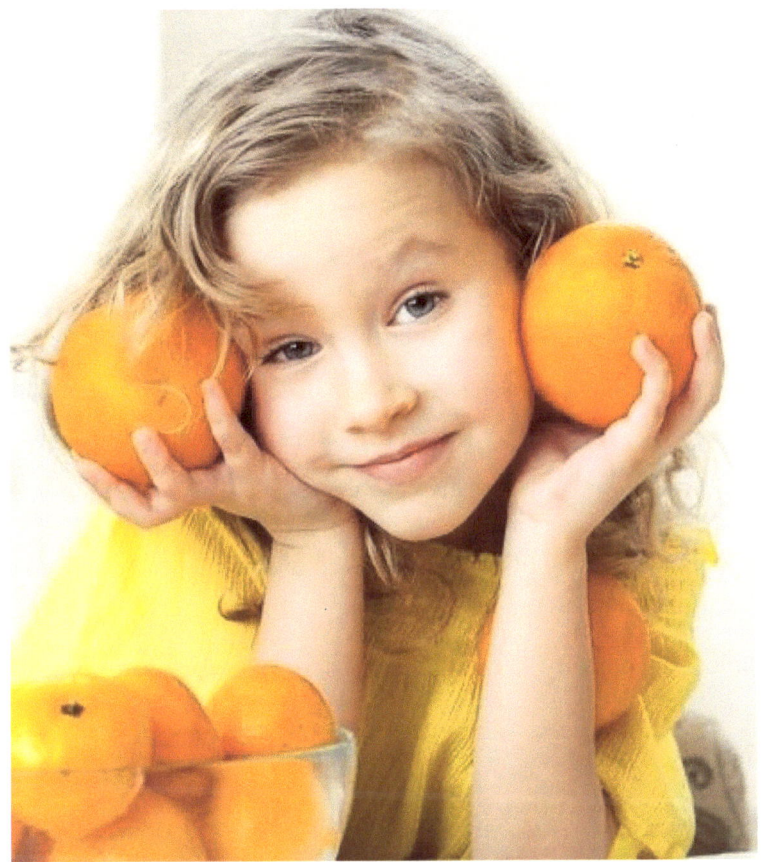

Oranges and lemons belong to the same citrus group as a slightly sour juicy fruit.

Lemon trees are very pretty and the lemon's flower is sweet/ but the fruit of the lemon is impossible to eat... That is what the flower children sang in the 60s. But the lyrics writer did not know that it was thanks to this impossible fruit, that sailors prevented themselves from suffering from scurvy at sea, rickety bones, loose teeth, and a weakened immunity system.

Once upon a time oranges and lemons were sold three for a penny, especially at Covent Garden, where the orange sellers, of which the most well-known is Nell Gwynn, used to sell these fruit to the theater goers every evening. These fruit also came in use, along with squishy and rotten tomatoes to pepper the actors on the stage, if the audience did not approve of their acting.

Oranges, Malta , Kinoo, and other citric fruit varieties are available all over the world. The best thing about these particular fruit is that you can eat and drink them everyday in every weather in moderate quantities and they are not going to give you any digestive problems.

In fact, with the coming of winter, you need to stock up on your store of fresh orange, and lemon juice drunk every morning so that you never suffer from cold, cough or any sort of winter related problems.

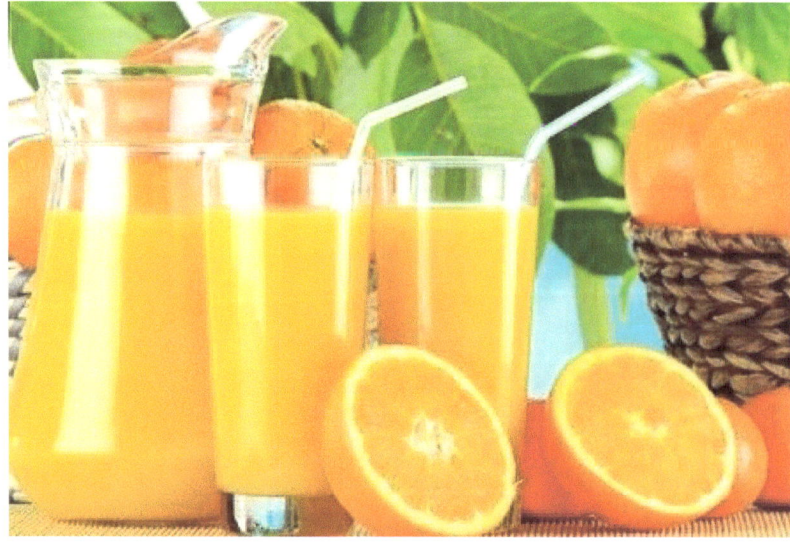

Even today, in many parts of the world, people start the day with a glassful of orange juice in order to refresh themselves. They would have been better off drinking plain water for all the good this concentrated stuff is doing them. However, if they are drinking real fresh orange juice, they are on the right track to good health and a healthy immunity system.

I had a friend who kept suffering from chronic cold, even when it was not the winter. All I thought it was possibly she was suffering from pulmonary problems like asthma and was reacting to pollen. So I just put her on a fresh orange juice diet with a little bit of lemon juice squeezed in it and a teaspoonful of honey and a little bit of fresh ginger juice for the next 15 days in order to see what happened.

Well, this was a trial run. And her colds vanished, never to appear again, so through trial and error, here is this excellent remedy, which you would want to implement on any member of your family, suffering from sniffles, cold, or even cough.

If you cannot bear it cold, especially in the winter, you can warm it, but just a little bit. Too much warming means all the vitamin C content is going to disappear into the wintry air. Try it out.

Oranges For Your Immunity System

In ancient times, oranges were fed in great quantities to all the citizens of the state, so that they never suffered from epidemics, especially in times of disease. This was normally done by mixing up orange juice with lemon juice to give the immune system more strength.

In many parts of Europe, where oranges did not grow, they were considered to be a delicacy for many centuries. In Queen Elizabeth's time, oranges were studded with cloves and used as a dry pomander by the nobility, in order to show two things – move out of the way, I am rich enough to afford oranges and spices, especially cloves.

Orange juice is excellent to rejuvenate you, especially when you are lethargic and feeling unenergetic. Also, if you are suffering from chronic insomnia, you may want to drink more orange juice. You may find yourself dropping off to sleep, naturally.

Heart Problems

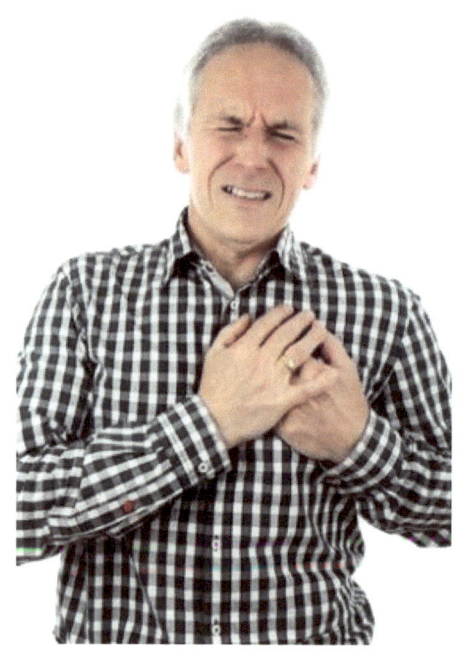

Oranges have been well known to prevent heart diseases since ancient times. For this, you needed to drink fresh juice of oranges regularly. It also prevents the arteries from constricting and thus causing a heart attack. If you are suffering from heart problems, you may want to try adding more orange juice in your diet. You are going to find a marked improvement in your state of health.

That is because the arteries are strengthened with the amount of vitamin C you are ingesting naturally through oranges. Also, they are going to get rid of all the accumulated cholesterol, and the toxic wastes present in your body, detoxifying your body, effectively.

Typhoid

I remember suffering from typhoid, once as a child, and the medicines were not doing me too much good. My grandmother immediately put me on fresh orange juice, with salt in it, because I was not being given solid food to eat. I survived. Thanks to this orange juice, my digestive system evened out, and was not harmed.

Within three months, I was back to eating heartily and eating again of all those items, which may have caused the disease to occur in the first place; but thanks to a strong immune system, I never got a typhoid attack again.

Asthma

People suffering from asthma and chronic cough should use this natural remedy, which is extremely effective. Take half part of orange juice and half part of warm water. To this add two hefty pinches of ground roasted cumin seeds, and three pinches of dried powdered ginger.

Give this to the patient two times a day until he is totally cured of asthma. It is going to take around a month for chronic cases and less than that for mild cases.

Pulmonary Pain

This normally occurs, if you have been out in the cold, without adequate protection. You find your rib cage area aching, because your lungs have frozen. So I am giving you this remedy, which you are going to do now, so that you have an adequate backup source for this winter.

Peel lots of oranges and dry them in the shade. That means, you are going to place them in a sunny corner of your home or garden, where there is a little bit of shade, but no direct sun, outdoors. When they are totally dry, crush them and put them in a glass bottle.

You have a very powerful winter remedy against pulmonary pain now. You are going to take three large tablespoons of this powder with warm water. Two doses and away goes that pain in the chest brought about through exposure to the harsh wintry elements.

Bloating

This may also occur if there is an infection in the stomach. This can be cured by taking 250 g of fresh orange juice, rock candy according to taste and 1 g of soda bicarbonate. Put the juice and the rock candy in water and make a sherbet. Now, squeeze the juice from the orange peel into this sherbet. Two – three drops is enough. Remember that the juice is rather bitter so do not squeeze in too much of the juice.

Now add the soda bicarbonate – edible soda – and while the mixture is still bubbling, drink it down. This is excellent for getting rid of edema in the stomach as well as jaundice. Do this every morning until you are cured.

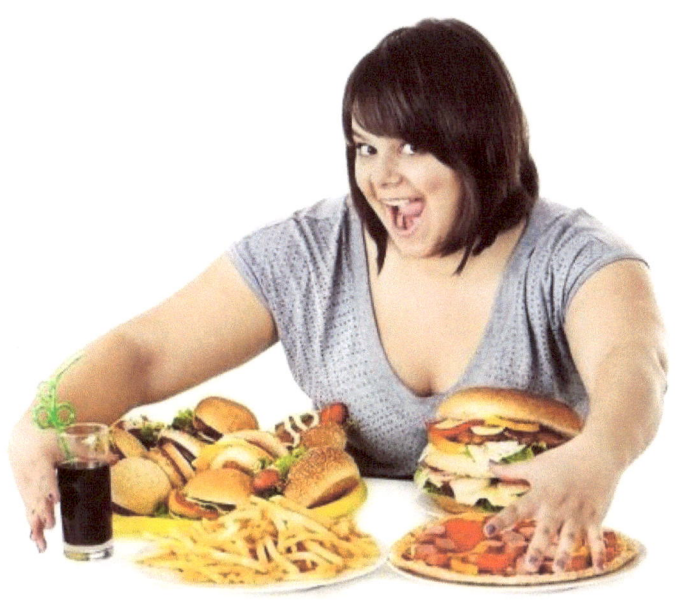

An unregulated diet is going to cause bloating.

Lemon Juice Cure

I was a very adventurous eater, as a child, thoroughly omnivorous. That is the reason why I often suffered from stomach ailments. But my grandmother would definitely not send me off to the hospital to be given plenty of toxic pills. Instead, I would be given the juice of one lemon in which she had mixed two hefty pinches each of black salt, roasted powdered cumin seed, 1 tablespoon full of honey and tell me to gulp it down.

This mixture was so delicious, that sometimes I did not need to feign a stomachache. According to her, this was an excellent drink to be drunk in the summer, to prevent dehydration, sunstroke and stomach problems.

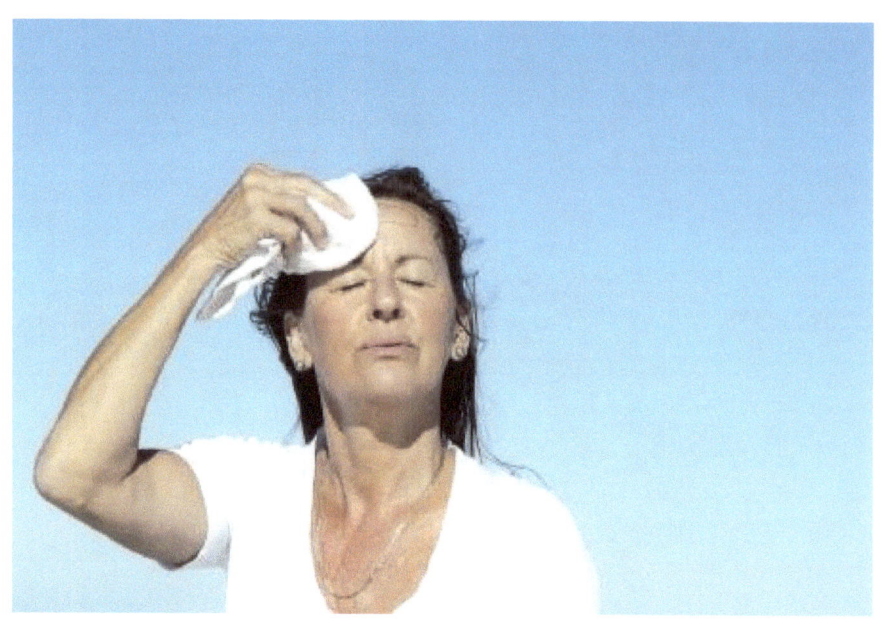

Also, this is something I did last night. I could not rest, because my throat had a tickle due to a wet cough, and I had begun feeling the start of a cold coming on, and a bit of fever, with the onset of the cold weather.

I got up and juiced one lemon in a glass of lukewarm water. In that I put 2 hefty pinches of black salt and pepper, and a few leaves of scissored mint. I drank it down, and after 15 minutes, I went to the drinks closet and got out 4 large tablespoons full of red wine. I normally do not drink any sort of drink with an alcoholic content, but this was for medicinal purposes and I did not have any brandy around. After drinking the wine, I diluted the alcoholic effect with a glassful of water.

After 20 minutes, and all the vestiges of fever, possible chest infection and cough and cold were gone. This morning, my breathing is easy, my nasal passages are clear, and I know that I am never going to suffer from any cold this winter as long as I have lemons with me followed with some red wine.

Traditionally, this lemon cure is done by taking out the juice of two lemons and putting it in boiling hot water. Allow the water to cool down, until it is lukewarm, and then add one teaspoonful of honey. This is drunk as soon as you are ready to go to bed and by tomorrow, you are definitely not going to have any signs of a cold.

Lemons for Your Teeth

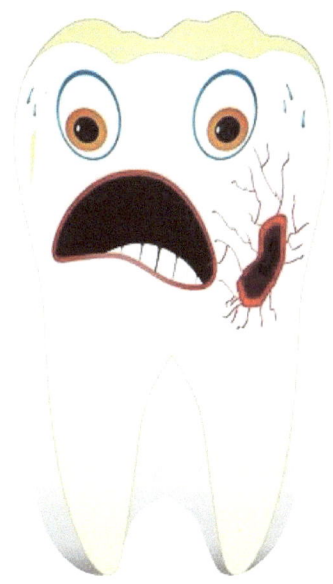

Since ancient times, lemon has been used as an excellent protective cure for teeth care. You could start with shade – dried lemon peel powdered with a little bit of salt and a little bit of soda bicarbonate. This is definitely the best teeth whitening agent, preventer of halitosis, and also prevents tooth decay.

When I was young, I saw a number of children who had never seen toothpaste before, having lived their lives in outposts of the Empire, using the natural way to clean their teeth, as their ancestors did before them. This was by taking half a lemon, dipping it in a solution of salt and mustard oil. Their teeth were whiter than Balsara pearls, against their dusky complexions and they never suffered from any sort of gum diseases like by bleeding of gums – gingivitis.

Even today, I have never needed to go to a dentist, because my teeth are in excellent condition and no way am I going to go there for whitening my teeth ever. I am just going to dip half a lemon in some salt and some mustard oil, and brush my teeth and gums with this mixture. Within four days, I am going to have teeth bleached out well and definitely not yellow, and also no teeth, mouth, and gum problems.

Anemia

If you find somebody suffering from a low blood count, anywhere in your vicinity, just start giving him the juice of one lemon and two tomatoes, fresh everyday. Along with that, you can give him the juice of one lemon with salt to taste. This helps in encouraging the red blood corpuscles to grow.

In olden times, people who suffered from less blood were given this treatment. The juice of one lemon was mixed in a glass of water with 25 g raisins. It was then placed over night in an airy place. The next morning, you would pick out the raisins from the lemon juice, and chew them, while drinking us a sip of lemon juice – water alternately.

The raisins helped in increasing the blood count, and giving you plenty of energy. It also help detoxify your body. In the same manner, if you have radishes around, you are never going to suffer from anemia just cut the radishes in bite-size pieces, mix with lemon juice and pieces of ginger. Eat this as a salad.

This will soon make you rosy with lots of healthy red blood in you.

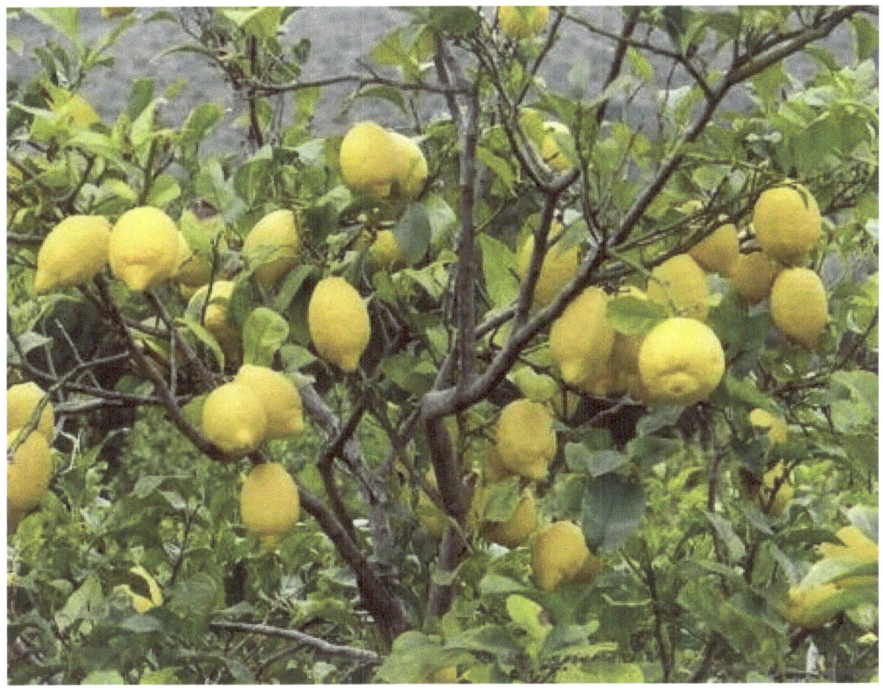

Remember, do not eat too many lemons, because that is also not too good for your body. The juice of two lemons is enough, when it is diluted with water. Raw lemon juice sprinkled on your food should never be more than one lemon.

Diarrhea

Diarrhea can be cured by just adding the juice of one lemon to a glass of milk. This prevents cramps, and if the diarrhea is accompanied with pain, then eat raw lemons without peeling them.

You can also add the juice of one lemon to a cup of water and drink it as often as you can. This is going to clear out your system. You are going to do this five times a day and by the next day, your diarrhea will have been under control.

If you do not want to drink it down, you can just put one drop of lemon juice in one spoonful of water, a little bit of salt and a little bit of sugar and drink this down five times a day. This is an extremely good electrolyte which will prevent diarrhea from dehydrating you as well as curing it.

You can also make this electrolyte with one cup of cold water in which you have mixed one fourth of a lemon and sugar and salt, according to taste. Drink this every two hours. Your diarrhea will be cured within the next 48 hours or before.

Toothache

Tooth ache normally strikes at midnight, especially when you do not have the dentist around. That is when you are just going to take some cloves and powder them. Add a few drops of lemon juice to the mixture and rub it all over the affected area. You are soon going to find that you may never need the ministrations of a dentist ever again.

Pimples

I never suffered from pimples, thanks to a very healthy childhood with plenty of exercise and extremely nourishing diet, without junk food and soft drinks, and that is why when at college, my friend suffered from pimples, they asked me for this remedy told to me by my grandmother.

Take 250 mL of boiled milk. Add the juice of one lemon to it. The milk is going to curdle, but do not worry, keep heating it until it is nice and thick and all the water has been evaporated. Allow it to cool, and then place it in a glass jar.

This is prepared in the morning, and applied in the evening, all over your pimples. You may want to prepare it fresh every day, if you have easy access to fresh milk, or you may use the product prepared before hand in your glass jar. Do this for about a week, and you are going to see your skin looking fairer and the pimples disappearing without any scars.

Gall Stones and Kidney Stones

In ancient times when there were no surgeons with state of the art technology around to get rid of gallstones and kidney stones for us, people had to resort to natural cures to get rid of these painful accumulations of Uric Acid.

To do this, you are going to take one lemon and mix it with rock salt. You are going to suck that lemon throughout the day. Do this as often as possible and you are soon going to find these stones dissolving and being eliminated through the elimination system.

Itching

Sometimes, you may find your skin itching due to dryness, or due to any other reason. Itching can grow tiresome, especially during the summer, when your skin is exposed to the rays of the sun, as well as it is suffering from prickly heat.

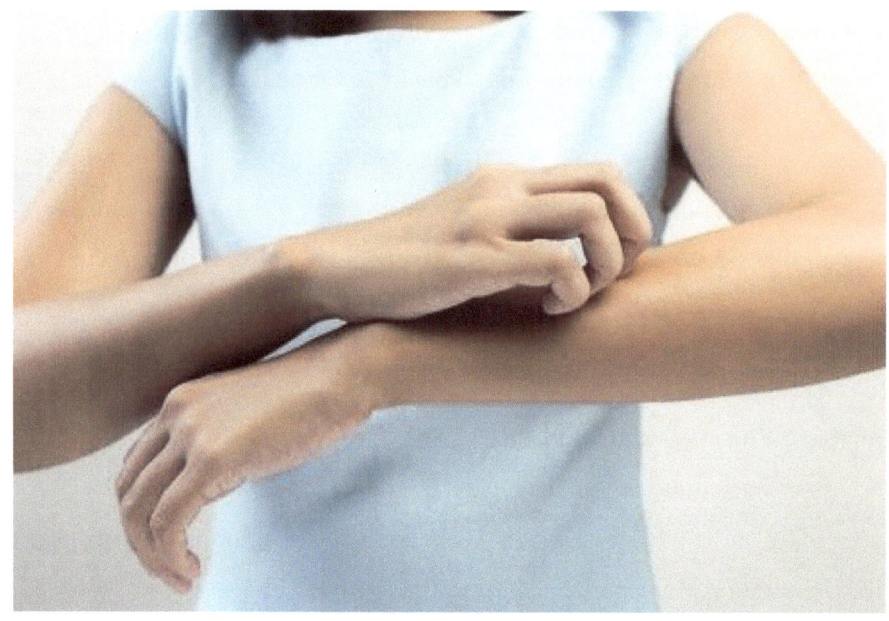

This could possibly be due to dry dehydrated skin...

For this, you are just going to put the juice of two lemons in your favorite oil – olive oil or coconut oil for choice. Allow it to cook on heat until the oil thickens. Put this in a glass bottle. You are going to massage this oil in all the areas affected by itching, three times a day, and you are going to see your skin glowing and itch free within the next three days.

Blackberries

We loved blackberries in blackberry pie, but many people do not know that these berries have been used since ancient times in native medicine. And because these blackberries are prolific only in the summer, and you cannot keep it for a long time in cold storage, this is the time when you are going to take full advantage of the blackberry juice and fruit.

Protection for Summer

This summer fruit has been made by nature to protect human beings from summer related problems, like sunstroke, heatstroke, and dehydration. Blackberries come in this category. The more blackberry juice you drink during this time, the lesser chances you will have of suffering from heatstroke or sunstroke.

Travel Sickness

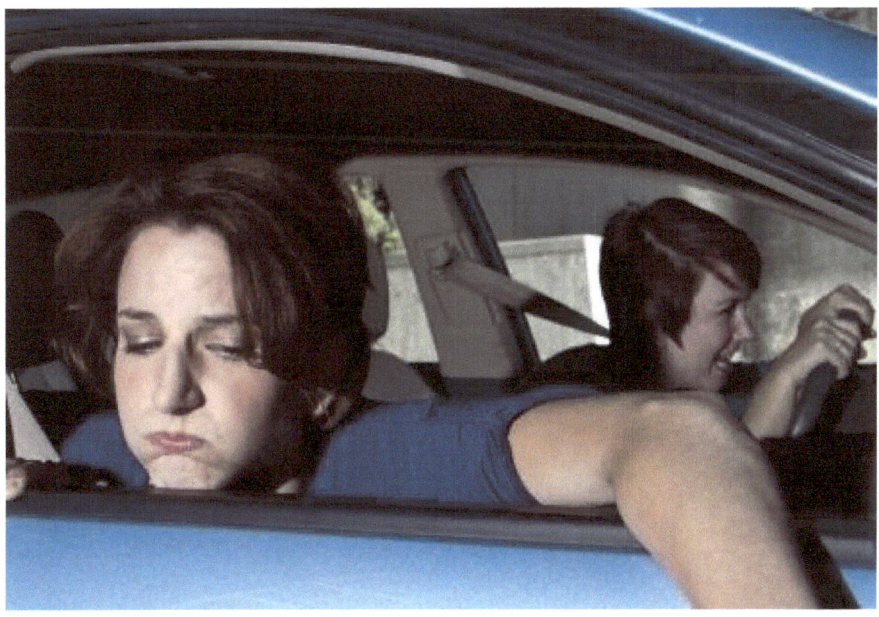

This is a remedy, a friend found out just by chance, and passed on to me. She suffered greatly from travel sickness, especially on a plane and in the car – poor lady – the moment the vehicle took off, she felt her system roiling in turbulent waves. Till one fine day, she found herself with a little box of blackberries, and began eating them in order to get her mind off the nausea accompanying the travel sickness.

Now she travels all over the world with blackberries in her cabin luggage, because she like Scarlett O'Hara says "As God is my witness, I will never go hungry again."

Diabetes

Blackberry seeds have been used since ancient times to cure diabetes. Just powder blackberry seeds, and put them in a glass bottle. You are going to drink a glass of water, in which 1/2 teaspoon full of powdered blackberry seeds have been dissolved, first thing in the morning. This is going to help improve your diabetes condition.

Blackberry juice has also been used for bringing down fever. Here, the ancients did not only drink it as a curative measure, but rubbed it on the hands, feet and soles as well as the body of a person who was feverish. This brought down the temperature and healed the sick patient.

Throat ailments

Powdered blackberry bark has been used to cure bronchitis, wounds in your throat, and asthma. This is a part of Native American medicine, where you made a decoction of powdered blackberry bark and powdered blackberry seeds in water. The decoction was made by putting these items in boiling hot water, and the water allowed to reduce itself to one fourth its quantity.

Drinking it down once a day until one was cured of bronchitis and asthma is an excellent way to get cured naturally.

Watermelons, Musk melons, and Cantaloupes

These of course come in my favorite summer fruit category. Eating these in large quantities all throughout the summer means that I am never going to be dehydrated, never suffered from a dry skin, because I rub the skin all over my face and hands, and feel energetic even in high-temperature zones.

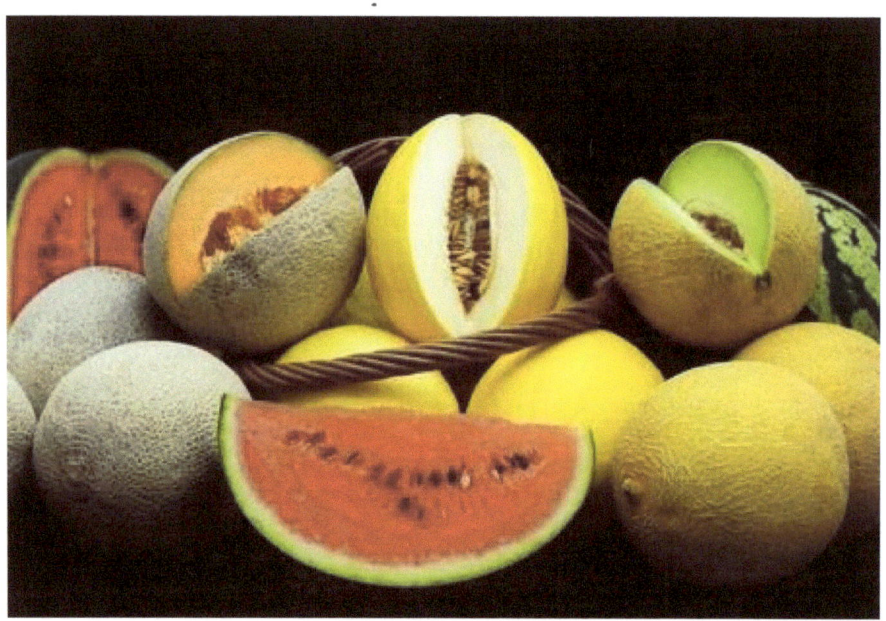

Musk melons, watermelons, and cantaloupes are never eaten on an empty stomach. Also, you are not going to drink any water, after you have eaten watermelon, because according to the elders, this was the easiest way to catch diarrhea or cholera.

Also, you are not going to drink any milk after you have eaten these fruit.

The best way to eat these fruit is to put them in cold water for a little while before you slice them up. This is going to take away the heating elements in the fruit's Constitution.

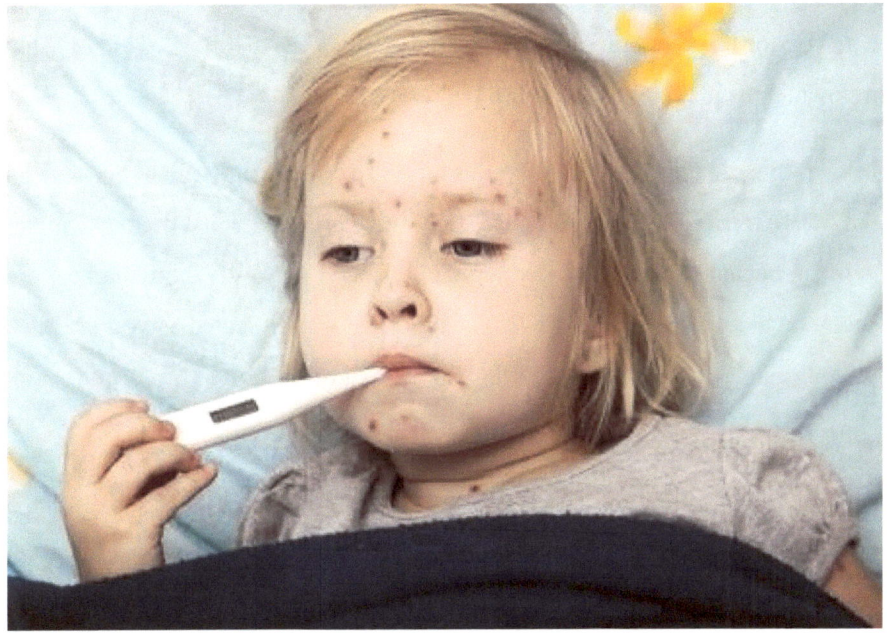

This infection could have been prevented if this little one's immune system was strengthened with a diet of grapes, oranges, watermelons, and other seasonal fruit.

Cholera is not a dreaded disease today, but once upon a time, it was an epidemic all over the world, making its appearance. Every summer, thousands of people died of cholera. Unless of course they were given this native remedy in order to help cure them.

That is why, the skins were dried in the shade, and powdered so that the people of the land had easy access to a cholera cure, whenever somebody said that the epidemic was abroad.

Take the dried skin of the musk melon – just two pinches of it, it is very powerful, and put it in 20 mL of your favorite alcoholic drink, brandy or whiskey for choice. Add 10 mL of water to dilute the alcohol content. Drink it down. This is going to help cure the cholera.

In fact, this remedy was very popular in the East with the British, because they were terrified of cholera. Also, they were great drinkers, men as well as women, because the climate demanded it. That is why everybody had easy access to alcohol, and taking a peg at sundown was expected as you lay back in your planter chairs and asked the "house – boy" to bring your drink.

These rough and tough men managed to get through the cholera epidemics every summer as long as their native bearers had musk melon skins drying in the shade.

Headaches

Watermelons were excellent for headaches. You just take some watermelon pulp, juiced it and added a little bit of rock candy to the mixture. This is to e drank, first thing in the morning, and you will never suffer from headaches. It also keeps you feeling energetic and fresh. Also, this juice was excellent for one reason that you would never suffer from excessive thirst, if you had watermelon juice in the morning.

Also, you can crush watermelon seeds with a little bit of water, and grind them really fine. When you have made a paste of this, you can apply this paste on the forehead of the person suffering from a headache. Along with curing this particular headache at this particular moment, it is also excellent for curing chronic headaches, if you continue this every day, until you are cured.

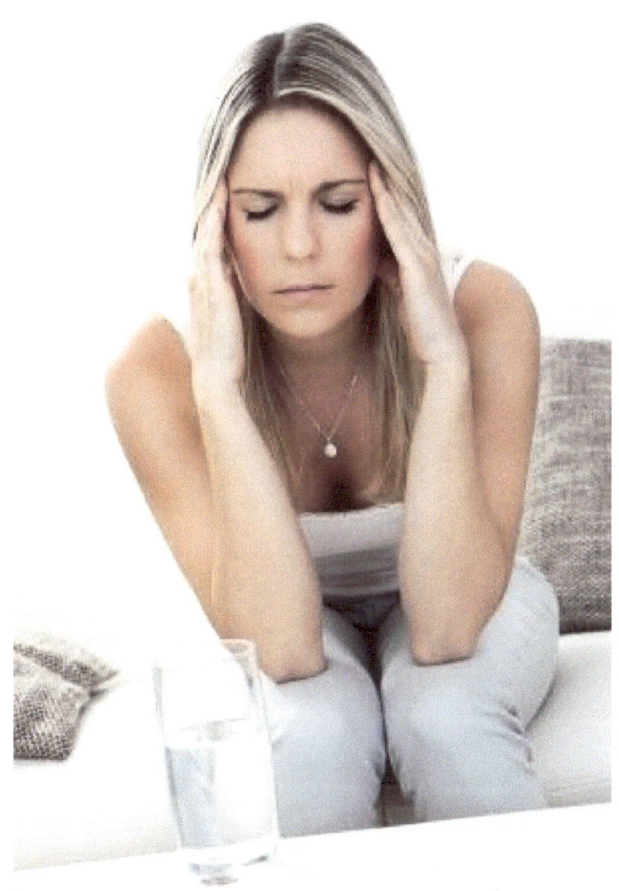

Hysteria, Neurosis, and Madness

Since ancient times, it was a well-known fact that people could fall into hysterical fits, maniacal fits, neurotic fits, and mad fits in the summer, and also often, if they were prone to such starts.

So instead of asking the village shaman to beat out the devils out of them with the help of neem twigs and burnt cayenne pepper fumes, the wise women of the village gathered together to feed that particular hysterical or neurotic patient 10 g powdered watermelon seeds, which had been soaked over night.

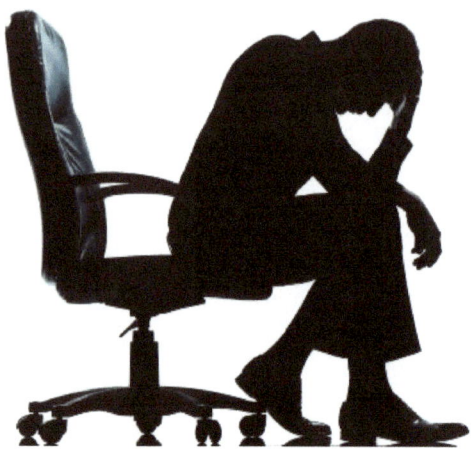

Stress, strain, and tension can often make a human being depressed and possibly feel hysterical because he thinks that things are getting to be beyond his control.

The next morning, they were ground together with 20 g of rock candy, 30 g of fresh butter, and four peppercorns. This was fed to the patient first thing in the morning. It was considered to be an excellent and permanent cure for madness, neurosis, hysteria, and mania.

Conclusion

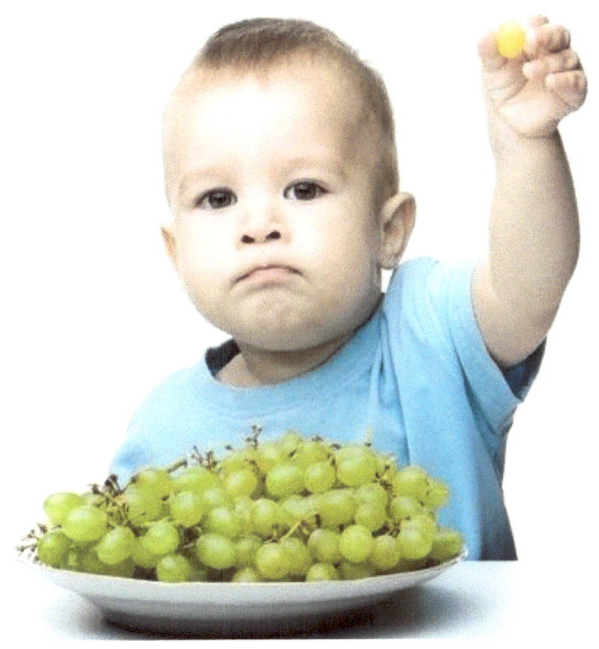

This book has given you plenty of information on how you can keep healthy, just by adding a larger quantity and helping of fruits in your daily diet. Fruits are the best shortcut to longevity, and good health.

Live Long and Prosper!

Author Bio

Dueep Jyot Singh is a Management and IT Professional who managed to gather Postgraduate qualifications in Management and English and Degrees in Science, French and Education while pursuing different enjoyable career options like being an hospital administrator, IT,SEO and HRD Database Manager/ trainer, movie , radio and TV scriptwriter, theatre artiste and public speaker, lecturer in French, Marketing and Advertising, ex-Editor of Hearts On Fire (now known as Solstice) Books Missouri USA, advice columnist and cartoonist, publisher and Aviation School trainer, ex-moderator on Medico.in, banker, student councilor ,travelogue writer ... among other things!

One fine morning, she decided that she had enough of killing herself by Degrees and went back to her first love -- writing. It's more enjoyable! She already has 48 published academic and 14 fiction- in- different- genre books under her belt.

When she is not designing websites or making Graphic design illustrations for clients , she is browsing through old bookshops hunting for treasures, of which she has an enviable collection – including R.L. Stevenson, O.Henry, Dornford Yates, Maurice Walsh, De Maupassant, Victor Hugo, Sapper, C.N. Williamson, "Bartimeus" and the crown of her collection- Dickens "The Old Curiosity Shop," and "Martin Chuzzlewit" and so on... Just call her "Renaissance Woman" - collecting herbal remedies, acting like Universal Helping Hand/Agony Aunt, or escaping to her dear mountains for a bit of exploring, collecting herbs and plants, and trekking.

Check out some of the other JD-Biz Publishing books

Gardening Series on Amazon

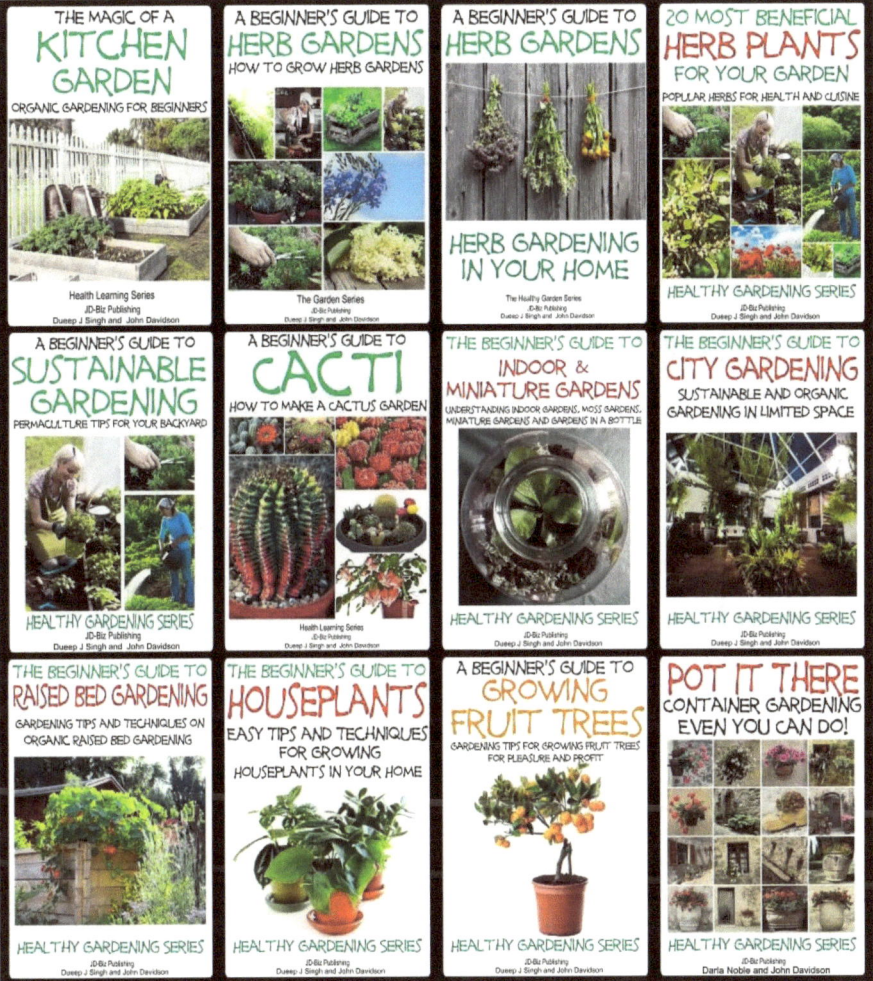

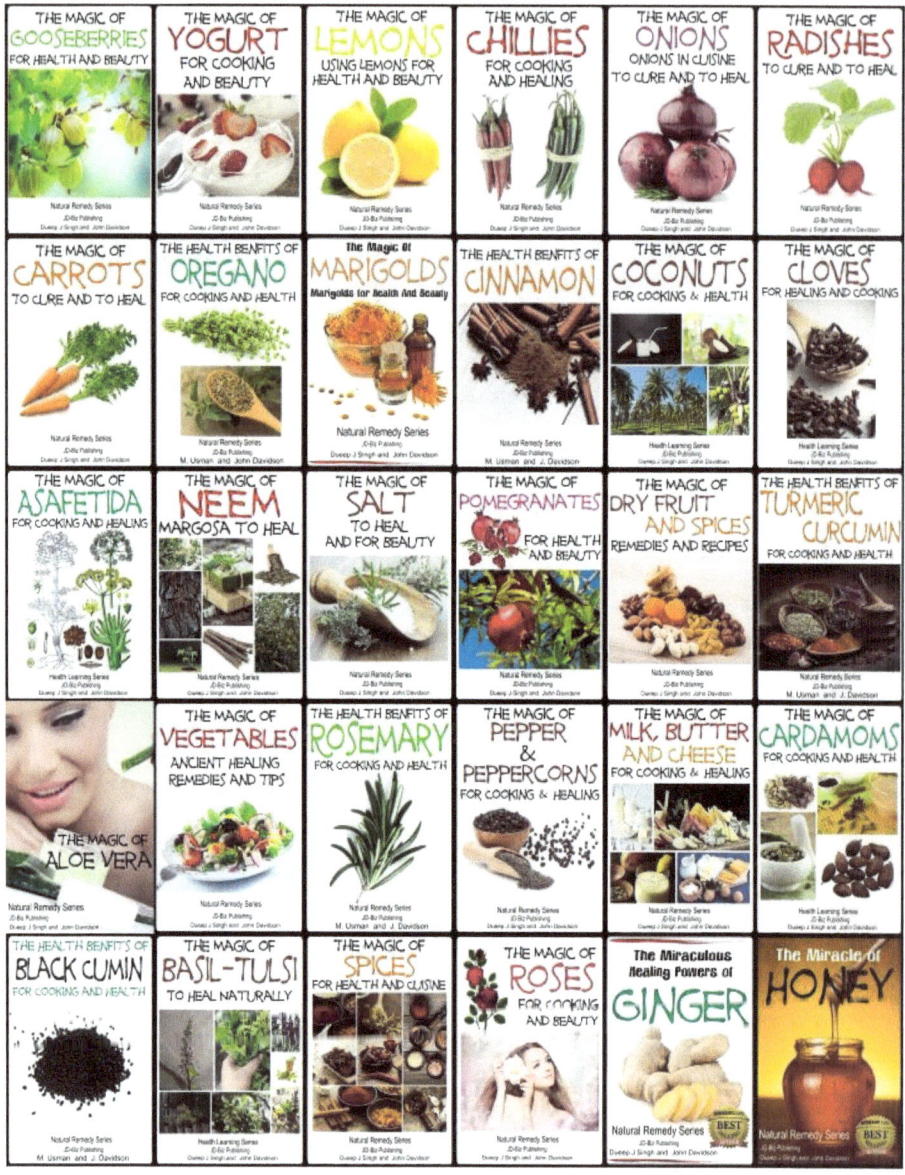

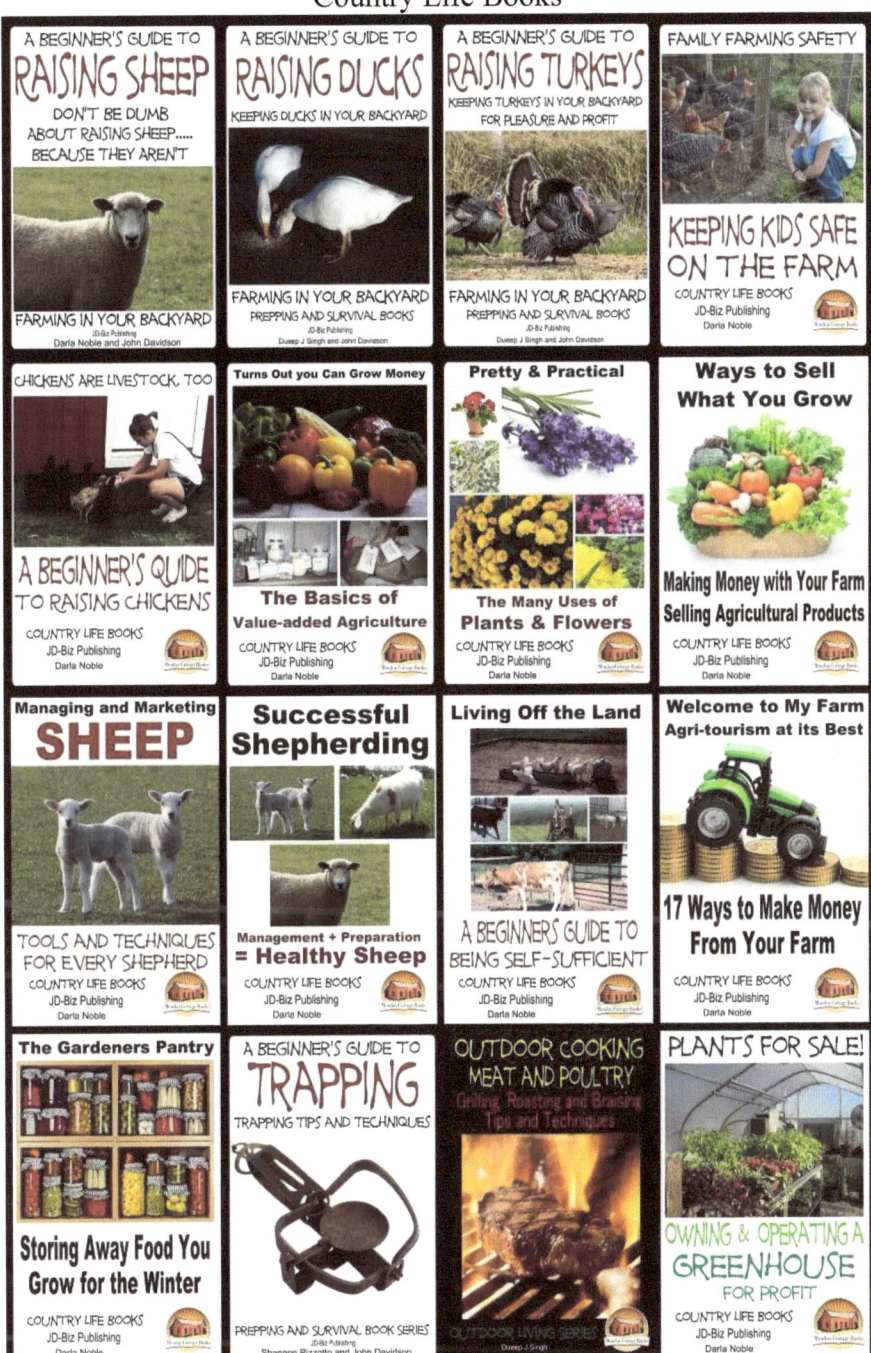

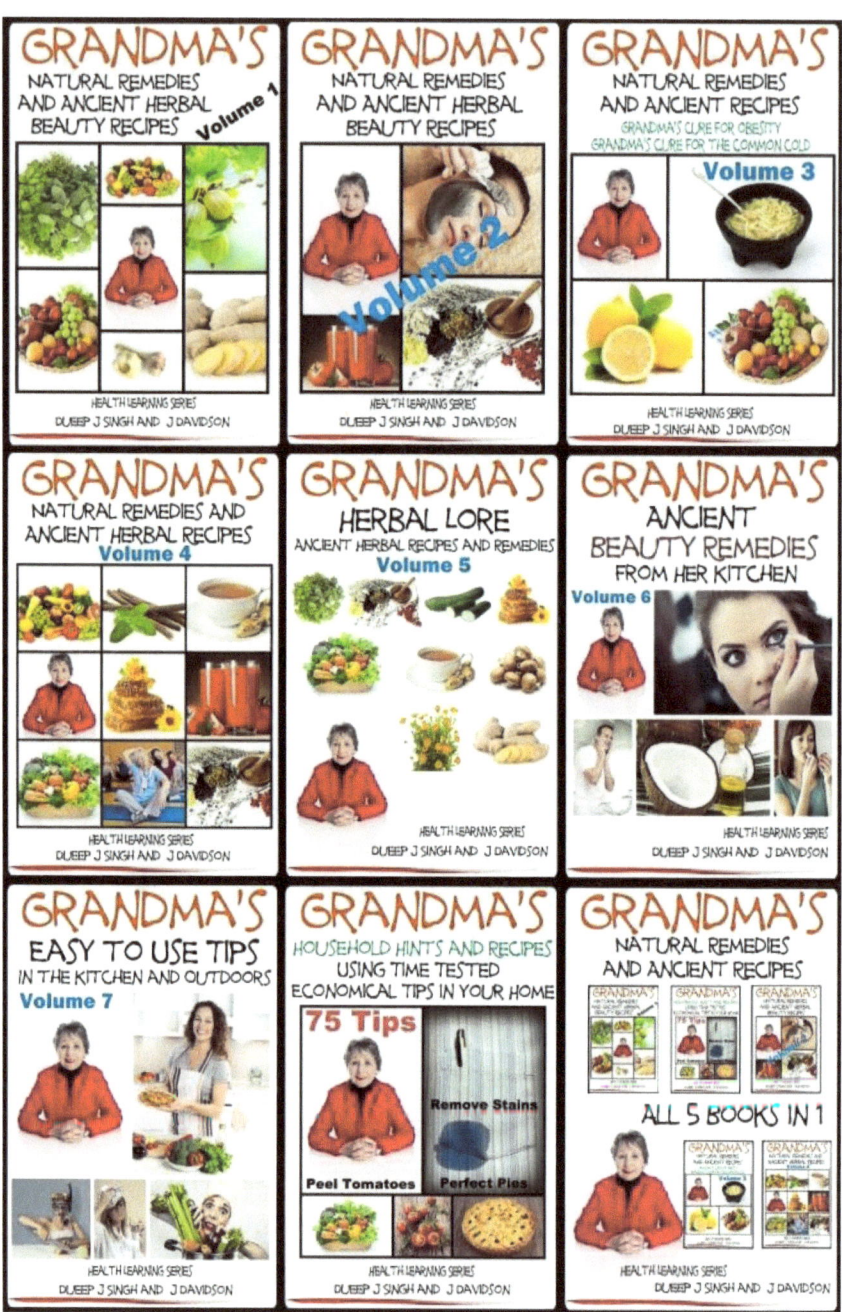

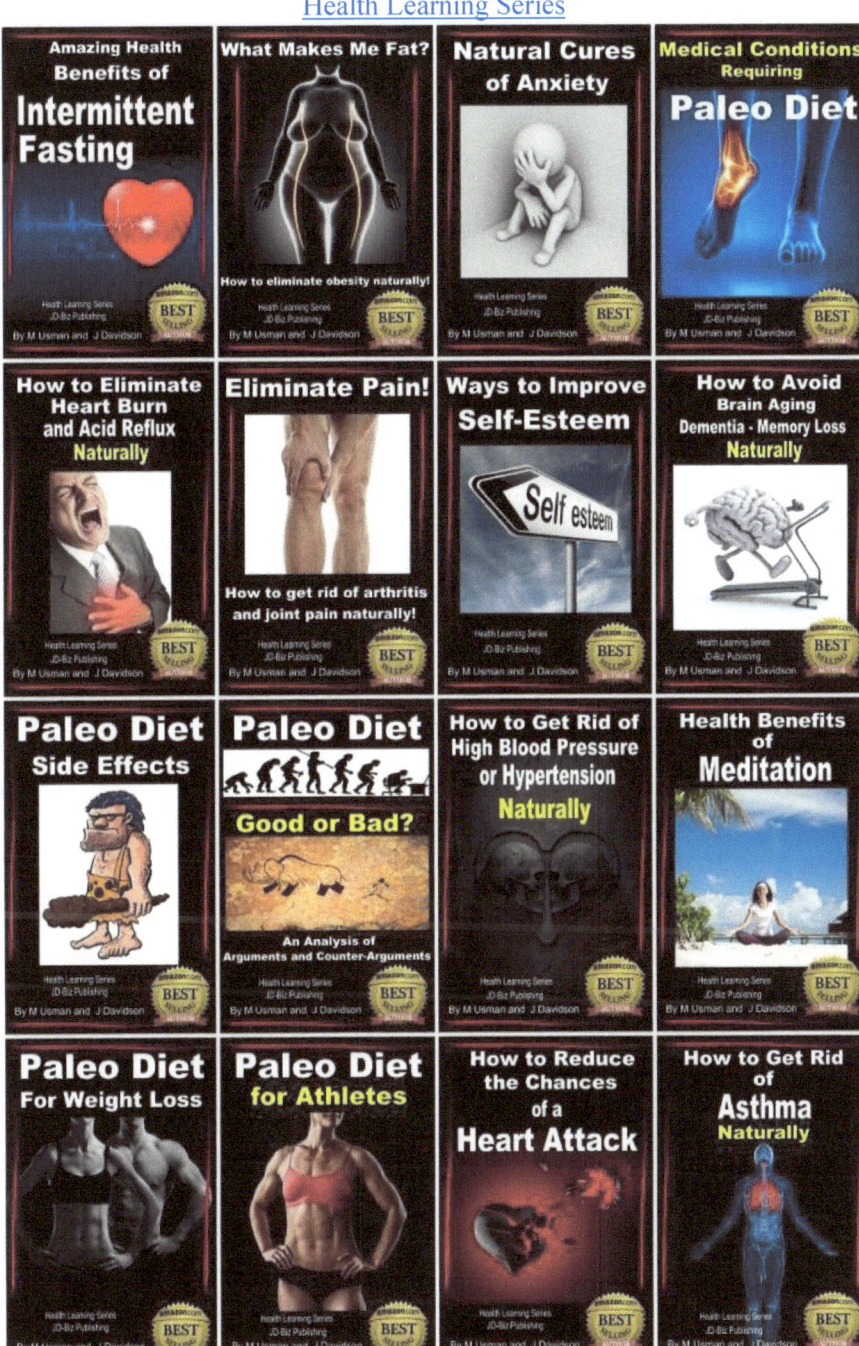

Amazing Animal Book Series

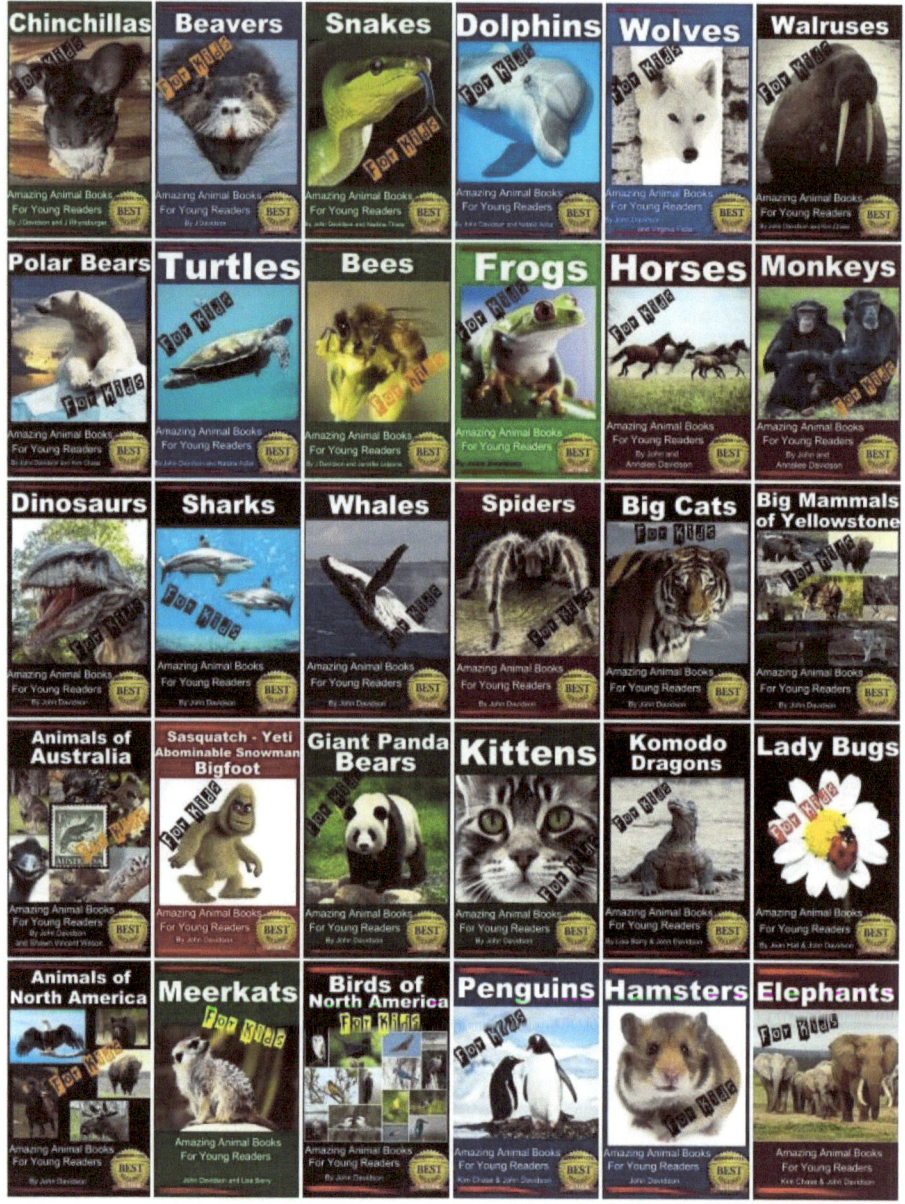

Learn To Draw Series

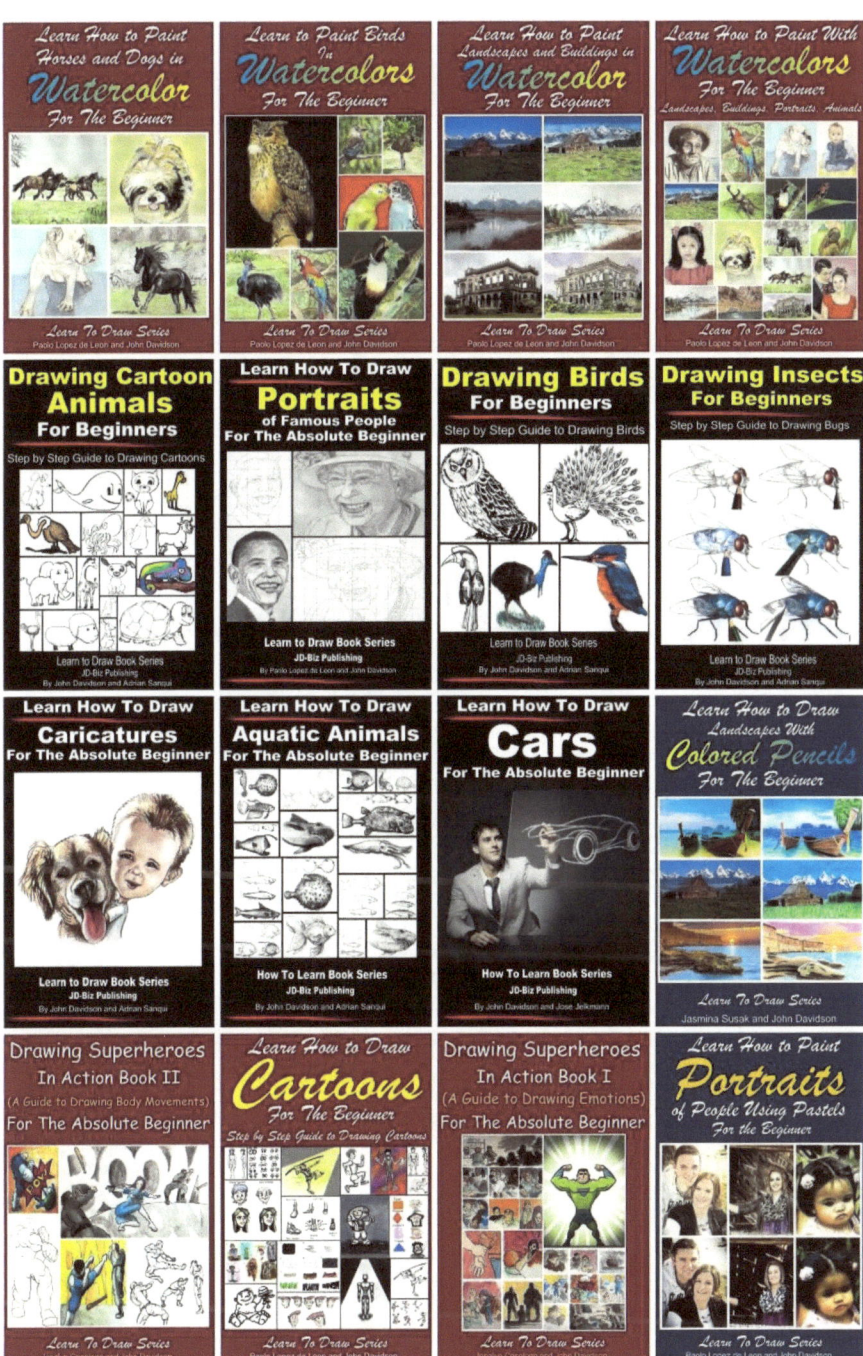

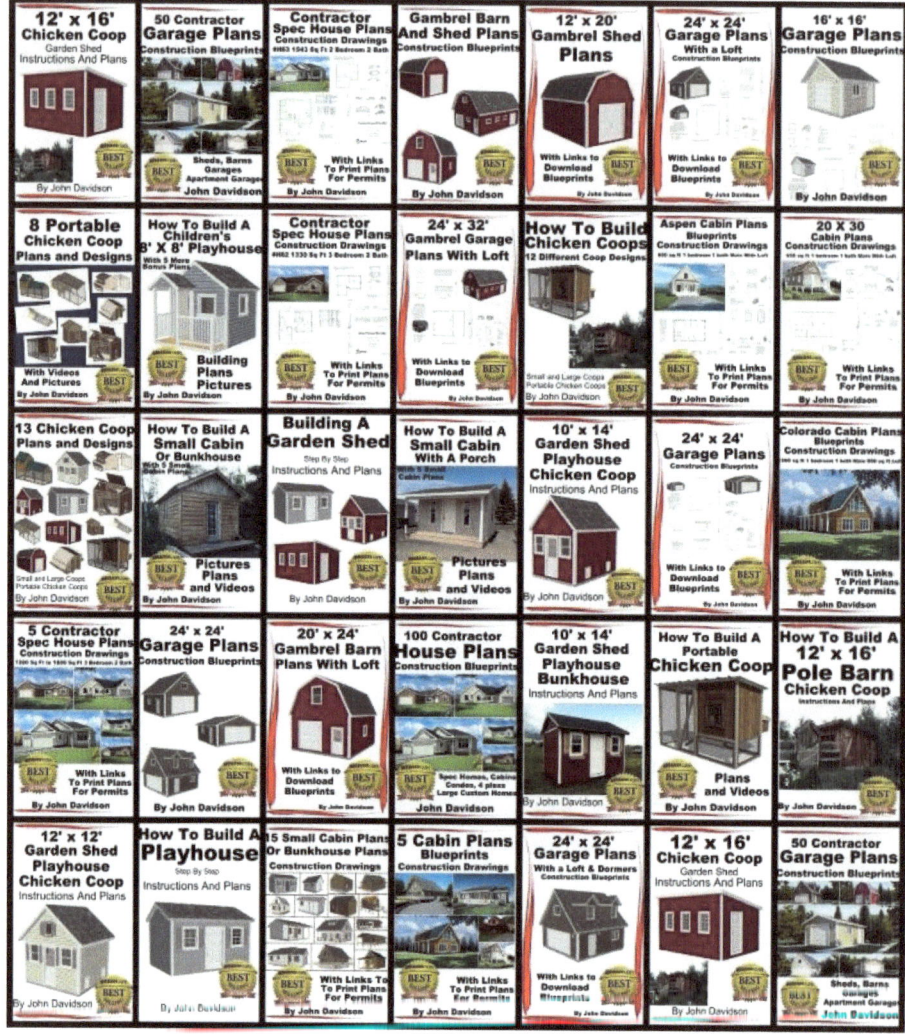

Entrepreneur Book Series

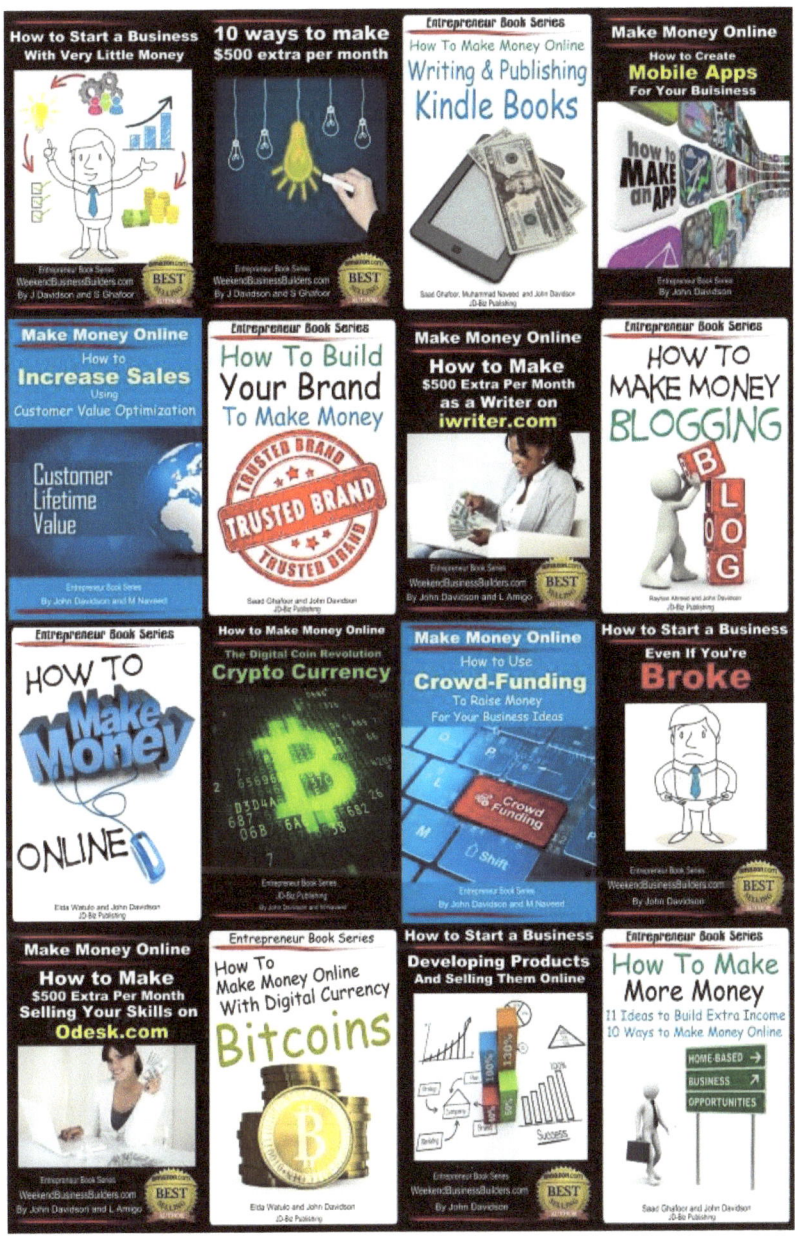

Our books are available at

1. Amazon.com

2. Barnes and Noble

3. Itunes

4. Kobo

5. Smashwords

6. Google Play Books

Download Free Books!

http://MendonCottageBooks.com

Publisher

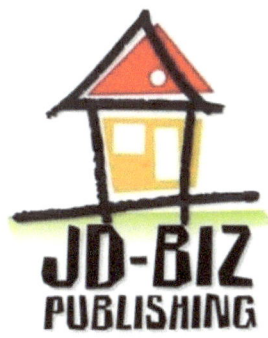

JD-Biz Corp

P O Box 374

Mendon, Utah 84325

http://www.jd-biz.com/

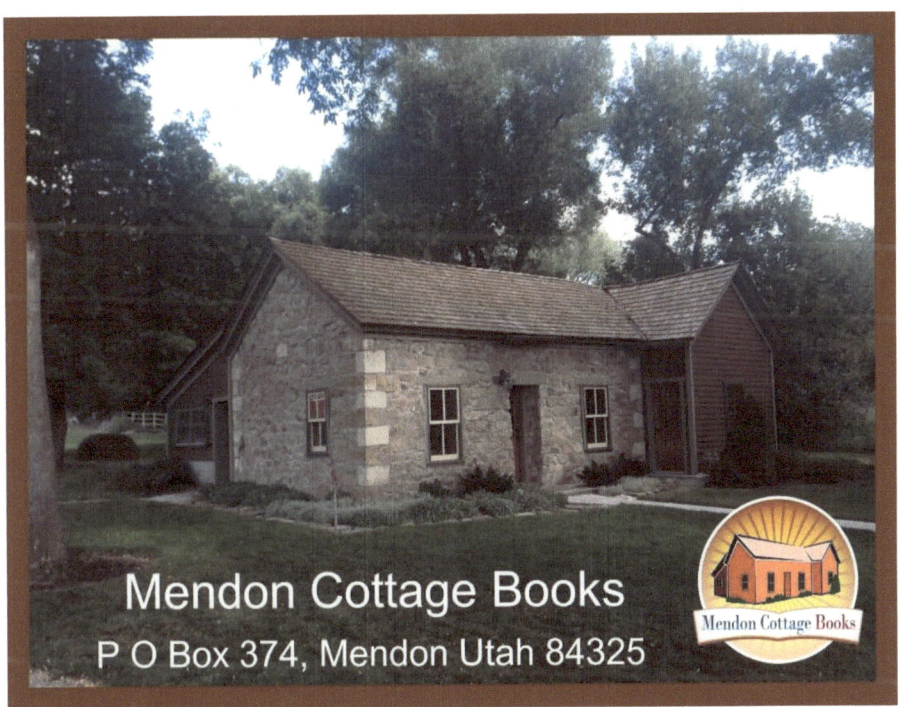

www.ingramcontent.com/pod-product-compliance
Lightning Source LLC
Chambersburg PA
CBHW050822290526
45792CB00001B/223